The No-BS Guide To IVF Medications

Unlocking Fertility Success: Simplifying Your Path to Pregnancy

By Jane Claire Aldridge

Copyright © 2024 Jane Claire Aldridge

All rights reserved. No part of this publication may be reproduced, distributed, or transmitted in any form or by any means, including photocopying, recording, or other electronic or mechanical methods, without the prior written permission of the publisher, except in the case of brief quotations embodied in critical reviews and certain other non-commercial uses permitted by copyright law. For permission requests, write to the publisher, addressed "Attention: Permissions Coordinator," at the address below.

Front cover image by Jane Claire Aldridge
Book design by Jane Claire Aldridge

Contents

Introduction 10
Chapter 1: Overview of IVF Medications 12
    Types of Medications associated with IVF 12
    Possible Side Effects of IVF Medications 13
        Side effects associated with IVF Medicines. 13
    How IVF Medications Are Administered 13
        Method of Administering IVF Medications 14
    Dosage and Timing: Getting It Just Right 14
    Injection Techniques: Making It Easier 15
    Managing Medication Schedules: Staying on Track 17
        Missed Doses: What to Do 18
    Cost and Accessibility: What You Should Know 19
    How Medications Interact: What to Keep in Mind 20
    Customizing Your Medication Plan: Tailored to You 20
Chapter 2: Hormonal Medications in IVF 23
    GnRH Agonists 23
        Function and Purpose 23
        Common Side Effects and Management Tips 24
    GnRH Antagonists 24
        Function and Purpose 24
        Dosage and Administration 24
        Common Side Effects and Management Tips 25
        Differences Between GnRH Agonists and GnRH Antagonists 26
    hCG (Human Chorionic Gonadotropin) 26
        Function and Purpose 26
        Dosage and Administration 26

- Common Side Effects and Management Tips 26
- Progesterone 28
  - Function and Purpose 28
  - Dosage and Administration 28
  - Common Side Effects and Management Tips 28
- Medication Overview Table 29
- Side Effects and Management Tips Table 29
- Medication Schedule Chart 30
  - CONCLUSION 31
- Chapter 3: Ovarian Stimulation Medications 33
  - Overview of Ovarian Stimulation and Its Importance in IVF 33
  - FSH (Follicle-Stimulating Hormone) 33
    - Function and Purpose 33
    - Dosage and Administration 34
    - Common Side Effects and Management Tips 34
    - Management Tips: 34
  - LH (Luteinizing Hormone) 36
    - Function and Purpose 36
    - Dosage and Administration 36
    - Common Side Effects and Management Tips 36
    - Management Tips: 37
  - Ovarian-stimulation medication table 38
  - Ovarian Stimulation Timeline 39
  - Additional Considerations 39
    - Monitoring and Adjusting Medications 39
    - Customizing the Treatment Plan 40
    - Ovarian Stimulation Process Table 40
  - Conclusion 41

Chapter 4: Supporting Medications in IVF ... 43
Overview of the Role of Supporting Medications in IVF ... 43
Antibiotics ... 44
Purpose and Use in IVF ... 44
Dosage and Administration ... 44
Common Side Effects ... 44
Side effects can include: ... 45
Management Tips ... 45
Steroids ... 45
Purpose and Use in IVF ... 45
Dosage and Administration ... 46
Common Side Effects ... 46
Management Tips ... 46
Thyroid Medications (if applicable) ... 47
Purpose and Use in IVF ... 47
Dosage and Administration ... 47
Common Side Effects ... 47
Management Tips ... 48
Supporting Medications Overview Table ... 49
Graph: The Role of Supporting Medications in IVF ... 50
Conclusion ... 51

Chapter 5: Managing Side Effects ... 53
Common Side Effects Associated with IVF Medications ... 53
1. Hot Flashes (Hormonal Medications, GnRH Agonists) ... 53
2. Mood Swings (Hormonal Medications) ... 54
3. Headaches (Hormonal Medications) ... 54
4. Bloating and Weight Gain (Hormonal Medications, Progesterone) ... 55

5.Abdominal Pain or Cramps (hCG, Progesterone) 55

6. Nausea (hCG, Progesterone)...56

Hormonal shifts can lead to nausea, making it difficult to keep food down or feel comfortable throughout the day. It is so important to feed your body highly nutritious food so nausea and vomiting can cause serious problems..56

Tip: Citrus & Mint Water 56

"Let's kick that nausea to the curb!" For nausea, try citrus-infused water with fresh mint leaves. Mint has a calming effect on the stomach, while citrus helps settle nausea. Simply add slices of lemon or orange and a few fresh mint leaves to your water. 56

Pro Tip: Keep ginger candies or ginger tea handy, as ginger is known for its stomach-soothing properties. Another important breathing exercise for nausea is to breath in through your mouth and exhale through your nose, in long deep breaths. 56

7.Injection Site Reactions (Progesterone)...56

Injection site pain, redness, or irritation is common with progesterone injections, and any other injections received during IVF. 56

Tip: Massage and Warm Compress 56

After your injection, give yourself some TLC. "A little post-injection massage never hurt anyone!" Gently massage the area to help the medication absorb better and reduce soreness. Apply a warm compress to ease any stiffness or tenderness. You can add the warm compress before you start feeling sore, right after your injection. It will help the medication absorb faster and reduce hard lumps....................56

Pro Tip: Switch up your injection sites regularly to avoid irritation or lumps. You can discuss different injection sites with your doctor. Also test the different sites and find places where you experience the least discomfort..56

8. Fatigue (Progesterone, Steroids)...57

Fatigue is common due to the hormonal changes induced by progesterone and steroids...57

Tip: Power Snack 57

"When you need a pick-me-up, go for a snack that packs a punch!" Keep energy-boosting snacks like Nut Butter & Banana Bites, or a trail mix of mixed nuts and dried fruit, on hand to keep your energy levels stable throughout the day. 57

Pro Tip: Incorporate mini-breaks throughout your day to rest. A quick 5-10 minute break can make a huge difference in recharging your batteries. Don't overdo it during this time. Be selfish with your time. For a couple of weeks try focusing on yourself, your mental health and the process. 57

9. Antibiotic Side Effects (Supporting Medications) 57

Guidance on When to Consult a Healthcare Provider 58

1. Severe Abdominal Pain or Cramps 58

2. Difficulty Breathing or Chest Pain 58

3. Unusual Bleeding or Spotting 58

4. Persistent or Severe Side Effects 58

5. Emotional Well-Being 59

Common Side Effects Management Table: 59

Frequency of Common Side Effects from IVF Medications 60

Conclusion 61

Chapter 6: Customizing Your Medication Protocol 63

Introduction to Personalized IVF Treatment Plans 63

Why Personalized Medication Protocols Matter 63

Factors That Influence Your IVF Medication Protocol 65

Age 65

Diagnosis 65

Previous IVF History 66

Tips for Discussing Your IVF Medication Protocol 66

Be Open and Honest About Your Health History 66

Ask Questions 67

Discuss Medication Timing 67

Inquire About Alternatives 67
How Your IVF Medication Protocol is Customized 68
Sample IVF Medication Protocol 69
Conclusion 70
Chapter 7: Effective Medication Management Strategies 72
Practical Tips for Tracking Medications and Schedules 72
    Create a Medication Calendar 73
    Tools for Organizing Medication 74
    Medication Management Apps 74
    Pill Organizers 75
Preparing for Injections and Oral Medications 76
    Injection Preparation Guide 76
Oral Medications: Tips and Preparation 77
Conclusion 78
Chapter 8: Additional Resources and Support 80
1. Resources for IVF Patients: Websites, Books, and Support Groups 80
2. Seeking Emotional and Informational Support 82
    Emotional Support 82
    Finding Reliable Information on IVF Medications 83
    Here's a quick checklist to evaluate sources: 84
Visual Resources: 84
    Reliable IVF Information Sources 84
Conclusion 86
Conclusion 88
Appendix 92
Disclaimer 95
About the Author 96

"You are not defined by your struggle, but by the hope and strength you carry through it."

Introduction

Going through IVF can feel like a wild ride. One moment, you're filled with hope, and the next, you might feel lost in a sea of information. But don't worry! This guide is here to help you make sense of it all. At the heart of IVF are all the different medications, and understanding them is key to your journey. Don't worry if you feel overwhelmed; this is normal. After reading this book, you will feel in control and empowered, and all these confusing medical terms will make complete sense.

So, what is IVF? In vitro fertilization, or IVF for short, is a fertility treatment that combines an egg and sperm outside the body—in a lab, to be precise. Easy, right? Nope, not at all. The books, pamphlets, and brochures make it sound so easy, but it isn't. And that's fine; it's a scientific marvel, not supposed to be easy, but it sure can be life-changing. When we gain the necessary knowledge about IVF, something complicated can become simple, and the puzzle pieces can easily shift into place in our minds. It offers hope to many people wanting to start a family, and that is incredible.

Once the embryos are created, medications come into play to help support the process—from getting your ovaries ready to preparing your uterus for the embryo. Each medication has its own job, working together to make the process as smooth as possible. Medications are a big part of IVF, and that is why I created this guide: to help you understand an essential part of the process.

Knowing about these medications is very important. Understanding the function, mechanism, and potential side effects of each medication can give you control during the process. This book is meant to be a helpful companion, offering support and breaking down complicated ideas into easily understandable information. You deserve clarity, and that is what this book delivers.

In the chapters ahead, we'll explore the different IVF medications. We'll cover everything from hormone treatments to supporting drugs. Each chapter is organized to give you clear explanations without confusing medical terms. Charts and graphs will help organize the ideas on the page and in your mind. Think of this book as a helpful map through the world of IVF medications, showing you the way with simple tips and advice.

So, grab a cup of your favorite tea, your markers for notes, and get comfortable. Let's start this journey together. Remember, you're not alone. You now have a friend, a companion to help you when things feel a bit overwhelming. Knowledge is your friend, and with it, you can face your IVF experience with confidence and peace of mind. Let's dive in!

Chapter 1: Overview of IVF Medications

Medications are a crucial part of the IVF process. From day one, it is very important that you are informed and up-to-date with your medications and responsibilities. Think of them as foundation builders—they ready your body, support each stage of the process, and enhance the possibility of a positive result. Every medication serves a distinct function, whether it's stimulating your ovaries to release several eggs or ensuring your womb lining is prepared to receive an embryo.

These aren't just random prescriptions; they're carefully selected and adjusted based on your unique needs. So, while the thought of taking medications can feel scary, knowing their role and how they work can help ease any worries. They're here to give you the best possible start on your path to parenthood.

Types of Medications associated with IVF

Type of Medication	Purpose	Examples	Key Notes
Hormonal Medications	Regulate fertility processes and egg maturation.	FSH (Follicle Stimulating Hormone), LH (Luteinizing Hormone)	Personalized to each patient's needs.
Stimulant Medications	Stimulate ovaries to produce multiple eggs.	Clomiphene, Gonadotropins	Increases egg quantity but doesn't guarantee quality.
Supporting Medications	Prepare the uterine lining	Progesterone, Estrogen	Creates an optimal

	for embryo transfer.		environment for implantation.

Possible Side Effects of IVF Medications

IVF medications are great scientific marvels, but any medication can have possible side effects. When we know what the possibilities are, we can better prepare ourselves for them. While these effects are generally temporary, it's important to understand what you might experience during your treatment and to know that your healthcare team is there to help manage any discomfort.

Side effects associated with IVF Medicines.

Type of Medication	Possible Side Effects/What to Expect
Hormonal Medications	Bloating, headaches, mood swings, and breast tenderness. These are usually temporary.
Stimulant Medications	Abdominal discomfort, ovarian cysts, mood swings, bloating, and weight gain.
Supporting Medications	Fatigue, breast tenderness, bloating, nausea, and mood changes.

How IVF Medications Are Administered

Now that we know the medications we're dealing with and their possible side effects, let's take a look at how these medications will be administered. This table explains the common methods of administering IVF medications. Understanding how each medication is given can help you feel more prepared and at ease as you navigate your treatment.

Method of Administering IVF Medications

Type of Medication	Method of Administration
Hormonal Medications	Typically administered through injections (subcutaneous or intramuscular). Some may be taken orally.
Stimulant Medications	Usually injected under the skin (subcutaneous) or sometimes into the muscle (intramuscular).
Supporting Medications	Administered via injections (usually subcutaneous), oral tablets, or vaginal suppositories.

Dosage and Timing: Getting It Just Right

As we have learned so far, IVF medications are divided into three groups. Each needs to be carefully monitored and administered at the right time and on the right days. Timing and dosage play a crucial role in IVF medication. Your doctor will provide a precise plan that's tailored to your body and needs. Adhering closely to this timetable is essential because the medications are intended to synchronize with your body's natural cycle. Think of the medication as dancers trying to mimic your body's natural rhythm.

Certain medications need to be taken at specific times during the day, while others may need to be taken multiple times. Make sure to carefully adhere to your schedule to ensure the effectiveness of the treatment, as missing a dose or taking one at the wrong time can have a negative impact. Don't let this stress you out or make you nervous; if you make any mistake, call your doctor and speak openly about it. Don't blame yourself for something before you know how serious it truly is. Most of the time, your healthcare provider will give you peace of mind in a few seconds, and you can adjust your schedule quickly according to their advice.

There are a few ways to help you during this process. I always think of myself as having two brains. One is for storing information about tasks that need to be finished quickly—everyday tasks. My second brain is my cell phone. I never want to overload my first brain; I want to give it rest and keep it fresh. So if there is anything during your IVF journey that you need to remember, take a few seconds to put it into your "second brain." This way, you have automated reminders that keep you accountable, and your "first brain" is available for all other tasks. A useful suggestion is to either set a daily alarm on your phone or maintain a record of your medication in a journal. In this manner, you can avoid needing to recall every detail and maintain focus without feeling overwhelmed. If you are ever unsure about timing, reach out to your doctor and jot down any timelines they provide.

Injection Techniques: Making It Easier

Now we reach the big one: the needles. I was so scared of any needle. If I had to draw blood, I would cancel my appointments. If I had to get a shot, I was miraculously healed that same day! I tried to avoid needles at all costs. But when it comes to IVF medications, it really isn't as bad as you think—and this comes from a true needle hater. Using injectable medications may seem daunting initially, but with some practice, it will become a regular part of your routine. Most IVF injections are administered subcutaneously or intramuscularly, as we learned earlier, with your doctor or nurse providing instructions on the proper technique when you begin treatment.

For subcutaneous injections, it's common to use the stomach or thighs, and it's important to switch up injection locations to prevent irritation. Before administering the injection, be sure to sanitize the area with an alcohol wipe and insert the needle at a 45- to 90-degree angle, considering the type of medication and your body's characteristics.

If you're nervous about giving yourself an injection, try to relax your muscles—don't tense up—and take a deep breath. Insert the needle as you exhale, blowing out the air in a long, relaxing exhale. Using ice before or after can help numb the area if the injection is painful. Some women may find it helpful to have a friend or significant other assist with the injections to increase comfort. My husband was a real champ with injections. The first few times, I just didn't have the courage, but after a while, it became easy—and I'm sure it will become easier for you, too. Keep your end goal in mind when injecting; this truly helped me. Temporary pain for eternal happiness—seems like a fair trade, wouldn't you say?

Remember, you have support from your healthcare team whenever you need additional tips or assistance. If you're ever unsure about anything, pick up the phone and call. Don't ever let yourself feel overwhelmed.

Managing Medication Schedules: Staying on Track

It may seem overwhelming to stay on top of your medication routine, but breaking it into easy steps can make it more manageable. Maintaining a well-organized system for taking multiple medications throughout the day is important as part of your treatment plan.

One effective method is to keep track of medications daily or use phone reminders. This way, you avoid relying solely on memory and can easily track each dose. Some women prefer to store their medications in a specific place, ensuring they're organized and accessible. When I was taking my medication, I created an Excel sheet that I kept on my phone and laptop. I jotted down the times and medications, and I made a checkbox for myself to ensure I took each dose and didn't forget anything.

Feel free to use this system for your journey. It makes medication tracking so much easier. Simply download it, fill in your times and any additional medications you're using. The check column is red, and each day you can change it to green or add a tick—whatever suits you best.

To access the Excel file, simply scan the QR code using your phone or tablet. Here's how:

1. Open your camera app on your smartphone.
2. Point it at the QR code (no need to take a picture).
3. A link will appear on your screen—tap the link to open it.
4. You'll be directed to the Google Drive file. From there, you can download the file.
   - On a phone, tap the three dots in the top right corner and select Download.
   - On a computer, click the Download icon at the top of the page.

Once downloaded, you can open and edit the Excel file on your phone or computer using an appropriate app like Microsoft Excel or Google Sheets.

If you have a schedule with several doses or timed injections, it's smart to anticipate any upcoming changes, such as travel or special occasions. If you're unsure about when or how to take a medication, be sure to consult your healthcare provider.

Missed Doses: What to Do

It happens—sometimes life gets in the way, and you might miss a dose. Don't panic! I know I'm saying this now, but when the time comes, panic may be all you do. If you realize you've missed one, the first step is to check your medication instructions or contact your healthcare provider for guidance.

In many cases, you can take the missed dose as soon as you remember, but if it's close to the time for your next dose, you may be advised to skip the missed one to avoid doubling up. It's important not to take extra doses to make up for a missed one without consulting your doctor first. It all depends on the timing and day of the missed dose. But remember, it's not the end of the world. Don't beat yourself up.

Cost and Accessibility: What You Should Know

The price of IVF drugs can be high, with overall treatment expenses varying depending on where you live, your insurance coverage, and the specific medications recommended. This is one of the biggest obstacles for most couples. Feeling worried about finances is normal, but there are resources available to help manage costs.

If you have insurance, consult your provider to determine coverage, as some plans may offer partial reimbursement for fertility treatments and medications. If there is limited or no coverage, ask your doctor or clinic about generic alternatives, discount programs, or payment options that could help reduce costs. So far, doctors have been very open about helping patients gain the necessary support to embrace the IVF journey.

Remember, your healthcare team is there not just to guide you through the medical side of IVF but also to help manage the financial aspects. Don't hesitate to have an open conversation with them about your concerns—it's a step toward finding the best options for your treatment and your budget. After exploring these options, you can choose one that works best for you.

If your budget simply doesn't allow for it and you're feeling as though all hope is lost, I want to assure you: it is not. There are many holistic methods we can explore to improve our chances of conceiving— things you may have never heard of. I have an upcoming book on how I turned things around with a holistic approach in a way I never thought possible. There is always hope, no matter what doctors or science may say. We, as women, know so little about our bodies, but goodness, we have an incredible and beautiful machine working for us.

How Medications Interact: What to Keep in Mind

It's important to understand how your IVF medications might interact with each other. In many cases, your doctor will carefully select a combination of medications that work together to give you the best chance for success. However, certain medications can have negative interactions that affect how well they work, so always make sure to share your full medical history with your healthcare team.

Inform your doctor if you are taking any other medications, such as those for thyroid issues or diabetes. Don't leave anything out. This will help tailor your IVF medication plan to avoid any adverse interactions. If you're uncertain about how your current medications may impact your IVF treatment, don't hesitate to consult your doctor or pharmacist for guidance. Maintaining clear communication ensures that everything works in harmony and that you're receiving the best possible treatment.

Customizing Your Medication Plan: Tailored to You

One of the wonderful aspects of IVF is that your treatment is customized specifically for you. Your healthcare provider will adjust the medications based on your unique needs, considering factors like your age, ovarian reserve, and any previous IVF treatments. This means that every IVF experience is different, and your medication plan will be specifically tailored to suit you. IVF is not a "one-size-fits-all" procedure—it's designed to give you special care that's in tune with your body.

Your doctor will guide you through any necessary changes, ensuring your treatment remains as effective and comfortable as possible. As you move forward, you'll be closely monitored, and your medication will be adjusted to reflect your body's responses. Trust in the personalized nature of your plan—it's designed to address your unique fertility needs.

"In the intricate dance of fertility, each medication is not just a step toward conception, but a reminder that even in the most delicate of moments, growth and new life are quietly taking shape."

Chapter 2: Hormonal Medications in IVF

Let's take a look at the second key type of medication used in IVF: hormonal medications. These medications play a crucial role in the IVF process by helping to control ovulation, prepare the uterus, and increase the chances of a successful pregnancy. Understanding the role of each medication in the carefully planned IVF regimen and knowing what to expect can help make the process more manageable. In this section, we'll explore the different types of hormonal medications, how they work, and important information about their use in IVF. Let's dive in.

GnRH Agonists

Function and Purpose

GnRH Antagonists are used later in the IVF process to prevent premature ovulation. In a typical menstrual cycle, your body releases a hormone that causes ovulation. GnRH Antagonists block this hormone, keeping the ovaries from releasing eggs too early. This gives your doctor full control over the timing of egg retrieval, which is crucial to successful IVF.

Dosage and Administration

GnRH Antagonists are typically injected subcutaneously once daily, beginning around day 5 or 6 of the stimulation cycle. The injections are short-term and only last for a few days before the egg retrieval process. You can schedule your injections on the free medication tracker found in Chapter 1. Your healthcare provider will explain the injection schedule in detail, and you will be given the necessary instructions to do it yourself at home.

Common Side Effects and Management Tips

Some common side effects include abdominal bloating, headaches, and mood swings. These are typically mild and go away after the medication is stopped. You can manage bloating by staying hydrated, eating light, healthy meals, and reducing salt intake. If headaches or mood swings are bothersome, let your doctor know, as they can help adjust your treatment or suggest additional ways to alleviate these issues. It is also important to remind yourself that you are undergoing hormonal treatment and emotional changes are possible, but manageable.

GnRH Antagonists

Function and Purpose

GnRH Antagonists are used in the later part of the IVF cycle to prevent the body from prematurely releasing an egg, also known as premature ovulation. This class of medication acts by blocking the signals that would normally tell the ovaries to release eggs, thereby keeping them in place until your doctor is ready for the retrieval. This control over timing is essential for IVF success because it ensures that eggs are retrieved at the optimal stage of maturation.

Dosage and Administration

GnRH Antagonists are generally given as a once-daily subcutaneous injection, starting around day 5 or 6 of the ovarian stimulation phase. This treatment is brief and typically only continues for a few days, right up until the egg retrieval procedure. Your healthcare provider will give you a detailed schedule for these injections, which you can record on the medication tracker provided in Chapter 1. They'll also guide you on the proper injection technique so that you feel comfortable administering them yourself.

Common Side Effects and Management Tips

Some common side effects of GnRH Antagonists include mild abdominal discomfort, headaches, and occasional mood shifts. Staying hydrated, eating balanced, low-sodium meals, and resting as needed can help ease bloating and discomfort. For headaches or significant mood changes, consult your doctor, as they can often suggest ways to manage these effects effectively. Remind yourself that these changes are temporary, and knowing how to manage them can help make the process smoother.

Differences Between GnRH Agonists and GnRH Antagonists

While both GnRH Agonists and GnRH Antagonists help control ovulation timing, they work quite differently. GnRH Agonists initially stimulate a surge in hormones before eventually suppressing them, requiring earlier administration in the cycle. In contrast, GnRH Antagonists work almost immediately to block hormone signals without causing an initial surge, so they are introduced later in the cycle. This direct suppression by Antagonists often makes them a more flexible option for preventing premature ovulation closer to egg retrieval.

hCG (Human Chorionic Gonadotropin)

Function and Purpose

hCG is a hormone that has a crucial function in the process of ovulation. It's used to trigger the final maturation of eggs before retrieval. The injection of hCG imitates the body's own hormone that initiates ovulation, but its timing is closely monitored by the doctor to ensure proper egg release.

Dosage and Administration

hCG is typically administered as a subcutaneous or intramuscular injection, around 36 hours before the scheduled egg retrieval. Your doctor will provide specific instructions regarding the timing and dosage of the injection, as well as whether a subcutaneous or intramuscular injection is best for your situation.

Common Side Effects and Management Tips

Bloating, tenderness at the injection site, and mild cramping are common side effects of hCG. These side effects usually go away after the egg retrieval procedure. If you experience cramping or tenderness, a heating pad or gentle exercise can help alleviate discomfort. If you notice more severe symptoms or signs of overstimulation, such as difficulty breathing or severe pain, contact your doctor immediately for further guidance. An ice compress is also recommended for tenderness at the injection site.

Progesterone

Function and Purpose

Progesterone is a hormone used to prepare the uterine lining for embryo implantation after egg retrieval and fertilization. After egg retrieval, your doctor will use progesterone to help thicken the uterine lining so it can support a fertilized embryo. Without adequate progesterone, the uterus may not be able to properly support pregnancy. Progesterone is so important in our natural cycle and that is why it is equally important in the IVFcycle.

Dosage and Administration

Progesterone can be administered via different methods: intramuscular injection, vaginal suppositories, or oral capsules. Intramuscular injections are commonly given daily after egg retrieval, while vaginal suppositories or oral tablets may also be part of your regimen. Your doctor will decide the best method based on your personal needs and response to treatment thus far. If you have any preferences feel open to make them known to your doctor.

Common Side Effects and Management Tips

Progesterone often causes bloating, breast tenderness, fatigue, and mood swings, as these are typical signs of early pregnancy. These symptoms are generally mild but can be uncomfortable. Using a heating pad for cramps, taking it easy when you feel fatigued, and being patient with mood swings can help manage these side effects. Although it can feel frustrating at times I like to think of it as hurdles to overcome before a final triumph. If the side effects feel overwhelming, talk to your healthcare provider for possible solutions. There is always a way to make the process more comfortable, so be open to ask. A hot bath and some down-time can also help to alleviate some discomfort and tenderness.

Medication Overview Table

Medication	Function	Dosage & Administration
GnRH Agonists	Suppresses natural hormones to control ovulation	Subcutaneous injection daily, sometimes long-acting options
GnRH Antagonists	Prevents premature ovulation	Subcutaneous injection once daily for several days
hCG	Triggers ovulation	Subcutaneous or intramuscular injection 36 hours before retrieval
Progesterone	Prepares the uterus for embryo implantation	Intramuscular injection, vaginal suppositories, or oral capsules

Side Effects and Management Tips Table

Medication	Common Side Effects	Management Tips
GnRH Agonists	Hot flashes, headaches, mood swings	Stay hydrated, practice relaxation techniques, use lubricants for dryness
GnRH Antagonists	Abdominal bloating, headaches, mood swings	Drink water, eat light meals, ask for help with symptoms if they worsen
hCG	Bloating, injection site tenderness, cramping	Use a heating pad, gentle exercise, contact your doctor if severe symptoms occur

| Progesterone | Bloating, breast tenderness, fatigue | Rest when needed, apply a heating pad for cramps, consult if side effects are scvere |

Medication Schedule Chart

To help you visualize how these medications fit into your treatment plan, here's a sample schedule for the medications used in a typical IVF cycle:

Day	Medication	Dosage & Administration
Day 1-3	GnRH Agonists	Daily subcutaneous injection
Day 5-6	GnRH Antagonists	Daily subcutaneous injection
Day 8-9	hCG	Single injection (36 hours before retrieval)
Day 5-10	Progesterone	Daily intramuscular injection or suppositories

This chart can help keep track of when each medication needs to be administered. The timing will be adjusted based on your personal cycle and response to medication, so always follow your doctor's specific guidance.

CONCLUSION

Knowing how your IVF medications work is crucial for maintaining a sense of control during the process. While it may appear overwhelming to manage, the assistance and advice from your doctor and healthcare professionals will ensure a seamless experience. From GnRH Agonists to Progesterone, each drug serves a distinct role in guaranteeing the success of your IVF cycle, and understanding what to anticipate can alleviate any worry or uncertainty. Bear in mind these details and keep in mind that you are not alone on this journey.

"The journey to new beginnings is never linear, but with each dose and each step, you are planting the seeds of hope for tomorrow."

Chapter 3: Ovarian Stimulation Medications

Ovarian stimulation is a key part of the IVF process that helps prepare your body for successful fertilization. Normally, in each monthly cycle, your ovaries release just one egg. But with IVF, we aim to retrieve multiple eggs to improve the chances of a successful outcome. To do this, special medications are used to "stimulate" the ovaries, encouraging them to produce more eggs.

Overview of Ovarian Stimulation and Its Importance in IVF

Ovarian stimulation medications help accomplish this by encouraging the ovaries to grow several mature follicles, each containing an egg.

The typical starting point is the use of gonadotropins (FSH and LH), which are hormones that promote the growth of follicles. Fertility specialists can manage ovary stimulation with these drugs to synchronize eggs for retrieval, ensuring ideal timing to retrieve all the matured eggs.

FSH (Follicle-Stimulating Hormone)

Function and Purpose

FSH is a hormone that occurs naturally and is crucial for the growth, development and maturation of ovarian follicles. It stimulates the ovaries to produce multiple follicles, each containing an egg, by encouraging the growth of the eggs. In IVF, artificial FSH is utilized to improve this procedure and support the growth of multiple eggs, boosting the likelihood of successful fertilization.

Dosage and Administration

FSH is typically given through a daily injection under the skin, typically beginning on the second or third day of your menstrual cycle. The dosage will vary depending on factors like your age, ovarian reserve, and how your body responds to the medication. Your doctor will modify the dosage according to blood tests and ultrasounds, closely monitoring the growth of your follicles.

Common brands of FSH include Gonal-F, Follistim, and Puregon. Each comes with specific instructions for how to mix and administer the injection, so be sure to follow your doctor's instructions carefully.

Common Side Effects and Management Tips

FSH is generally well-tolerated, but some women may experience side effects. These can include:

- Ovarian hyperstimulation syndrome (OHSS): This is a condition characterized by swollen and painful ovaries, possibly due to excessive egg development. Although uncommon, it can be severe, therefore stay vigilant for signs like stomach bloating or discomfort. Always contact your healthcare provider if you are unsure of any symptoms or feel severe discomfort.
- Headaches and mood swings: Like other fertility drugs, hormonal shifts can lead to mood swings. It is important to take care of you mental health, so be sure to take some much needed rest and engage in relaxing activities that bring you peace.
- Injection site reactions: It is common to experience redness, swelling, or pain at the site where the injection was given.

Management Tips:

- Keep your body hydrated and steer clear of salty foods in order to reduce bloating.

- Practice relaxation methods such as deep breathing or yoga to control mood fluctuations. You can experiment and try different activities that bring you peace. Try painting, cooking, walking or any other recreational activities. I love arts and crafts and hiking.
- Apply ice or use a warm compress for injection site discomfort. You can use a warm compress before feeling discomfort and give yourself a head start.

LH (Luteinizing Hormone)

Function and Purpose

LH is another hormone that plays a role in the final stages of follicular development and ovulation. In IVF, LH is often combined with FSH or administered alongside it to ensure that the follicles mature properly. While FSH helps to stimulate the growth of the follicles, LH supports the final maturation of the eggs within those follicles. The combination of these two hormones enhances the chances of having multiple eggs ready for retrieval at the same time.

LH is often administered in combination with FSH as part of a combined medication regimen. This dual approach mimics the natural hormonal fluctuations that occur in a typical cycle, helping to coordinate the timing of ovulation and egg retrieval. So far we can see how important it is that we mimic the natural bodily processes with these medications. They are here to give us that extra boost, but they are simply copying what our bodies try to do naturally

Dosage and Administration

LH can be administered through subcutaneous injections, similar to FSH. In some cases, a combination medication containing both FSH and LH is used, which may simplify your medication schedule. The dosing schedule is individualized based on your response to the medications.

Brands like Menopur or Repronex are commonly used, as they combine FSH and LH in one injection. Your doctor will determine the exact dosage based on your response to ovarian stimulation.

Common Side Effects and Management Tips

The side effects of LH are similar to those of FSH, though some women may notice specific reactions related to the medication combination. These can include:

- Headaches, bloating, and abdominal discomfort: Similar to FSH, these side effects can occur as the ovaries respond to the medication.
- Mood swings and irritability: As we know hormonal fluctuations can affect emotions.

Management Tips:

- Rest and relaxation can help manage mood swings. Don't put unneeded stress upon yourself during this time. Take a few weeks to focus on the process and focus on yourself. You are allowed to be selfish.
- If bloating or abdominal discomfort is significant, reduce your salt intake and increase fluid consumption, always keep a water bottle with you. It will encourage you to sip through the day.
- Watch for signs of ovarian hyperstimulation syndrome (OHSS), especially if more than 20 follicles develop. Keep your doctor up to date on any discomfort.

Ovarian-stimulation medication table

Medication	Function	Dosage & Administration	Common Side Effects	Management Tips
FSH (Follicle-Stimulating Hormone)	Stimulates follicle growth and egg production	Daily subcutaneous injection, adjusted based on monitoring	OHSS, headaches, mood swings, injection site reactions	Hydrate well, avoid salty foods, relax to manage mood swings
LH (Luteinizing Hormone)	Supports follicle maturation and ovulation	Subcutaneous injection, often combined with FSH	Headaches, bloating, abdominal discomfort, mood swings	Rest, reduce salt, increase fluids, manage stress

Ovarian Stimulation Timeline

Here is a SAMPLE medication schedule for ovarian stimulation in a typical IVF cycle, incorporating FSH and LH medications. THIS IS SIMPLY A SAMPLE, IT SHOULD NOT BE FOLLOWED.

Day	Medication	Dosage & Administration
Day 2-3	FSH (Follicle Stimulating Hormone)	Daily subcutaneous injection
Day 5-6	LH (Luteinizing Hormone)	Daily subcutaneous injection (if using a combination drug)
Day 8-10	FSH and LH	Adjust dosage based on response to ultrasound and blood work
Day 10-12	Trigger shot (hCG)	Administer 36 hours before egg retrieval

This table represents the timeline for typical medication usage in IVF. However, the exact schedule may vary depending on your individual cycle and response to medications.(Please remember to follow your specific schedule, given by your healthcare provider)

Additional Considerations

Monitoring and Adjusting Medications

Ovarian stimulation medications require careful monitoring throughout the IVF cycle. Your doctor will regularly perform ultrasounds and blood tests to track how your ovaries are responding to the treatment. The goal is to stimulate the ovaries without over-stimulating them, which is why your medication dose may change during the cycle based on these results.

Customizing the Treatment Plan

Your treatment may differ from others depending on your age, ovarian reserve, and any previous IVF cycles. While FSH and LH are the main players in ovarian stimulation, other medications may also be included to support your specific needs. Always communicate openly with your doctor about any concerns or symptoms you experience.

Ovarian Stimulation Process Table

Stage	Action	Purpose	Outcome
FSH Administration	FSH (Follicle-Stimulating Hormone) injections	Stimulates the ovaries to grow multiple follicles	Follicle growth begins, increasing egg count
LH Administration	LH (Luteinizing Hormone) injections	Finalizes the maturation of the developing follicles	Follicles reach full maturity, ready for retrieval
Egg Retrieval	Eggs are collected from mature follicles	Prepares mature eggs for fertilization	Eggs are retrieved and stored for fertilization

Conclusion

Ovarian stimulation is one of the most critical parts of IVF, as it increases the number of eggs available for fertilization, maximizing your chances of success. By using medications like FSH and LH, your fertility doctor can guide the development of multiple eggs in a controlled and precise way. While the process can be overwhelming at times, understanding the role of these medications and knowing what to expect can help you feel more empowered and prepared for the journey ahead. Keep in mind that your treatment plan will be customized to fit your individual needs, and your healthcare team will provide you with ongoing support and guidance. Just like that we have reached the end of Chapter 3. I believe that all the puzzle pieces are starting to fall into place for you. Let's move on to the next important step which is the supporting medicines in IVF.

"In the process of creating life, patience becomes your strongest ally, and understanding the medicine that nurtures you can transform uncertainty into empowerment."

Chapter 4: Supporting Medications in IVF

While ovarian stimulation medications like FSH and LH are critical to egg development in IVF, supporting medications play an essential role in ensuring that the process runs smoothly. So what is supporting medications? These medications support various bodily functions—such as immune health, hormone regulation, and infection prevention—that can impact the outcome of IVF. They are like tiny warriors ready to face any problems that may arise. In this chapter, we'll explore some of the common supporting medications used in IVF, including antibiotics, steroids, and thyroid medications, and how they contribute to the success of the treatment.

Overview of the Role of Supporting Medications in IVF

Supporting medications help to create an optimal environment for egg retrieval, fertilization, and embryo implantation. While they are not the primary medications for stimulating egg production, they help manage any underlying conditions and prepare the body for a successful IVF cycle. In other words not all women will use them and they are simply there to give extra support in certain areas where it is needed.

These medications can:

- Prevent infections during egg retrieval and embryo transfer.
- Support immune function, as a strong immune system is crucial in fertility.
- Regulate hormones like thyroid hormones, which can affect ovulation and embryo implantation.

Antibiotics

Purpose and Use in IVF

Antibiotics are commonly prescribed to prevent infections during IVF. This is especially important before and after egg retrieval, as the procedure involves inserting a needle into the ovaries to collect the eggs. Antibiotics help reduce the risk of bacterial infections, which could interfere with the process.

Commonly prescribed antibiotics during IVF include doxycycline and azithromycin. They are typically administered just before and after the egg retrieval procedure to prevent infection.

Dosage and Administration

- Doxycycline: Typically taken orally in the days leading up to and following the egg retrieval procedure. Dosage may vary based on the specific protocol but often starts with one pill daily for 3-5 days. Your doctor will discuss the specifics with you and you should follow the instructions given by him. The dosages may vary from woman to woman.
- Azithromycin: Often given as a single dose (oral), typically the day before or the day of egg retrieval. Your doctor will discuss the specifics with you and you should follow the instructions given by him. The dosages may vary from woman to woman.

Common Side Effects

Antibiotics are generally well-tolerated, but some women may experience side effects. Remember to always discuss allergies or any intolerances with you doctor ahead of time.

Side effects can include:

- Gastrointestinal issues: Nausea, diarrhea, or upset stomach.
- Yeast infections: Antibiotics can disrupt the natural balance of bacteria in the body, leading to yeast overgrowth. (Some doctors might prescribe probiotics to combat this side effect.)
- Skin reactions: Rashes or sensitivity to the sun. Ask your doctor about these possibilities and protect yourself from the sun when going outside.

Management Tips

- Take antibiotics with food to reduce gastrointestinal discomfort.
- Stay hydrated, and maintain a healthy diet to avoid yeast infections.
- Use sunscreen to protect sensitive skin, as antibiotics can increase sun sensitivity.

Steroids

Purpose and Use in IVF

Steroids, specifically prednisone or dexamethasone, are used in some IVF protocols to suppress the immune system and prevent inflammation. These medications can help improve the chances of embryo implantation, especially in women with certain autoimmune conditions. Steroids are thought to reduce immune responses that may interfere with embryo implantation, promoting a more favorable environment for the embryo to implant in the uterus. Just like we discussed before it is important to create a "happy home" for the embryo to thrive.

Dosage and Administration

Steroids are typically administered orally, with doses being adjusted based on individual needs. The usual dosage starts at a higher level, which is gradually tapered off as the IVF process progresses. For each individual dosages will vary and specific protocols prescribed by the doctor should be followed.

- Prednisone: Often started at 5-10 mg daily, then gradually reduced.
- Dexamethasone: Can be prescribed at 0.5-1 mg daily, tapered down based on the IVF protocol.

Common Side Effects

While steroids can be highly effective, they also come with some potential side effects:

- Weight gain: Steroids can cause fluid retention and increase appetite, leading to temporary weight gain.
- Mood swings: Some women may experience irritability or emotional changes.
- Increased blood sugar: For those who are sensitive, steroids can raise blood sugar levels, which may require monitoring. (Speak to your doctor if you have any blood sugar issues or if you are diabetic)

Management Tips

- Manage weight gain by following a healthy, balanced diet and staying active. Small adjustments like going for a walk can make a big difference during this time.
- Practice stress-reducing techniques like mindfulness, journalling or yoga to help with mood swings.
- Monitor blood sugar levels, especially for women with diabetes or prediabetes.

Thyroid Medications (if applicable)

Purpose and Use in IVF

Thyroid health plays a significant role in fertility. An underactive thyroid (hypothyroidism) or an overactive thyroid (hyperthyroidism) can disrupt ovulation and hinder embryo implantation. Therefore, regulating thyroid hormones is important in IVF.

If you have problems with your thyroid, your doctor might give you medications such as levothyroxine (for low thyroid function) or methimazole (for high thyroid function) to maintain thyroid balance while undergoing IVF treatment.

Dosage and Administration

- Levothyroxine: This is a popular drug for hypothyroidism, usually taken once a day. Blood tests are used to determine the ideal thyroid hormone levels and adjust the dosage accordingly. (For each individual it will be different)
- Methimazole: It is typically prescribed once a day for hyperthyroidism, with the dosage determined based on thyroid function. (For each individual it will be different)

Common Side Effects

Thyroid medications are generally well-tolerated, but side effects can occur:

- Levothyroxine: Taking too much can lead to symptoms of hyperthyroidism, such as weight loss, rapid heartbeat, or anxiety.
- Methimazole: Common side effects can include skin rashes, stomach upset, and, rarely, liver issues.

Management Tips

- Regular blood tests to monitor thyroid levels and adjust medication as needed.
- Take thyroid medication on an empty stomach for better absorption.
- Report any unusual symptoms, like fatigue or mood swings, to your doctor.

Supporting Medications Overview Table

Medication	Purpose	Dosage & Administration	Common Side Effects	Management Tips
Antibiotics (Doxycycline, Azithromycin)	Prevent infections during egg retrieval and embryo transfer	Oral doses before and after egg retrieval	Gastrointestinal upset, yeast infections, skin reactions	Take with food, stay hydrated, use sunscreen
Steroids (Prednisone, Dexamethasone)	Suppress immune system to promote embryo implantation	Oral doses, tapered down after initial higher dose	Weight gain, mood swings, increased blood sugar	Eat balanced meals, stay active, monitor blood sugar levels
Thyroid Medications (Levothyroxine, Methimazole)	Regulate thyroid function for optimal fertility	Oral daily medication, adjusted based on thyroid blood tests	Weight changes, heart rate issues, stomach upset	Monitor thyroid levels, take on an empty stomach, report symptoms

Graph: The Role of Supporting Medications in IVF

Below is a simple pie chart illustrating the relative roles of different medications in the IVF process:

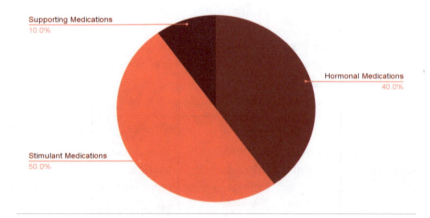

This breakdown shows that while the majority of medications in IVF are related to hormonal and stimulant medications, supporting medications still play a critical role in optimizing the environment for successful fertilization and embryo transfer.

Conclusion

Supporting medications are very important in ensuring the best possible outcome, in certain scenarios. These medications and some others might be prescribed by your doctor. I always encourage women to make a list of any previous health problems when going for their initial appointment, be open about any problems or concerns you have or any medical problems that you have had in the past. Nothing is too small, if you can remember it then tell your doctor about it. This way you know that you have given the doctor all the possible information and he can make the best recommendations to suit your specific story. While they do not directly influence egg production, they help regulate immune responses, prevent infections, and support overall hormonal balance, all of which create the best environment for implantation. By understanding how these medications work, their potential side effects, and how to manage them, you'll be better prepared for the IVF process. Always consult with your doctor about the specific medications in your treatment plan, as each individual's needs can vary. Be open, be honest and don't be afraid to ask questions.

"Each medication is a small but powerful piece of the larger puzzle, helping to shape a future that begins with faith and unfolds with strength."

Chapter 5: Managing Side Effects

Receiving IVF treatment requires the use of different medications, as we know. Some may occasionally result in side effects. As we've progressed through the chapters so far, we've touched on some of the side effects and how to manage them. In this chapter, we will dive deeper. I will help you find easy ways to manage discomfort and give you the smoothest, problem-free experience possible. The discomforts can vary from mild and temporary to more noticeable symptoms. Knowing what to anticipate and how to handle side effects is essential for maintaining control throughout your experience. In this chapter, we will explore ways to handle side effects and offer advice on when to seek help from your healthcare provider.

Common Side Effects Associated with IVF Medications

The side effects vary depending on the medication you are using, but they are usually easy to control. Here is a summary of the typical side effects linked to IVF drugs.

1. Hot Flashes (Hormonal Medications, GnRH Agonists)

- **Hot Flashes (Hormonal Medications, GnRH Agonists)**

    Hot flashes can be a common issue, especially with medications that suppress or stimulate hormones. While you can't entirely prevent them, there are ways to cool down quickly and feel more comfortable.

- **Tip: Cold Compress for Your Neck**

    "I know you're already bringing the heat, but let's cool you down before you turn into a walking sauna!" Place a cold compress or a damp towel behind your neck when a hot flash hits. The skin at the back of your neck is rich in blood vessels, and cooling it down can help your body regulate temperature faster. Keep a small spray bottle in the fridge with a few drops of peppermint or lavender oil for an instant cool-down spritz.

- **Pro Tip:** Keep a chilled face mist or cooling gel handy throughout the day for a quick refresher.

2. Mood Swings (Hormonal Medications)

Fluctuating hormone levels during IVF can lead to mood swings, making it harder to stay emotionally balanced and feel positive about the process.

Tip: Relax with Aromatherapy

When emotions feel like they're on a rollercoaster, try calming scents like lavender or chamomile essential oils. Diffuse them around your space for a peaceful environment.

Pro Tip: Keep calm and take deep breaths. If you're feeling overwhelmed, take a few minutes to practice deep breathing or a quick 5-minute meditation. You'd be surprised at how much a short break can reset your emotional compass!

3. Headaches (Hormonal Medications)

Headaches are a common side effect of IVF medications due to hormonal fluctuations.

Tip: Peppermint & Lavender Oil Relief

"Let's not let this headache drive you mad!" Apply a few drops of peppermint and lavender essential oils (mixed with a carrier oil like coconut or almond oil) to your temples, forehead, and the back of your neck. Gently massage to relieve tension and ease headache discomfort. Peppermint improves circulation, while lavender has soothing properties.

Pro Tip: Drink plenty of water, because dehydration can make headaches worse. Hydrate with citrus-infused water to give your body a refreshing, natural boost!

4. Bloating and Weight Gain (Hormonal Medications, Progesterone)

Hormonal treatments, especially progesterone, can cause bloating and fluid retention, leading to discomfort.

Tip: Hydrate with Peppermint & Lemon Water

Feeling bloated? "Let's flush that out, shall we?" Drink peppermint and lemon-infused water to promote digestion and reduce water retention. Add a few sprigs of fresh peppermint, slices of lemon, and cucumber to your water and let it sit for 10 minutes.

Pro Tip: Keep a stash of healthy snacks like trail mix (with nuts and dried fruit) or Nut Butter & Banana Bites nearby to snack on throughout the day. Small, balanced meals help minimize bloating and keep you energized.

5. Abdominal Pain or Cramps (hCG, Progesterone)

Some discomfort is common as the body adjusts to the hormonal effects, especially around the time of the embryo transfer.

Tip: Gentle Yoga Stretches

Feel the cramping coming on? "Take a deep breath and stretch it out." Gentle yoga poses, like Child's Pose or Legs Up the Wall, can help promote blood flow and ease discomfort. It's like giving your body a hug from the inside!

Pro Tip: Heat pads or warm compresses can provide comfort for abdominal pain. Just make sure it's not too hot—your skin deserves the gentle touch!

6. Nausea (hCG, Progesterone)

Hormonal shifts can lead to nausea, making it difficult to keep food down or feel comfortable throughout the day. It is so important to feed your body highly nutritious food so nausea and vomiting can cause serious problems

Tip: Citrus & Mint Water

"Let's kick that nausea to the curb!" For nausea, try citrus-infused water with fresh mint leaves. Mint has a calming effect on the stomach, while citrus helps settle nausea. Simply add slices of lemon or orange and a few fresh mint leaves to your water.

Pro Tip: Keep ginger candies or ginger tea handy, as ginger is known for its stomach-soothing properties. Another important breathing exercise for nausea is to breath in through your mouth and exhale through your nose, in long deep breaths.

7. Injection Site Reactions (Progesterone)

Injection site pain, redness, or irritation is common with progesterone injections, and any other injections received during IVF.

Tip: Massage and Warm Compress

After your injection, give yourself some TLC. "A little post-injection massage never hurt anyone!" Gently massage the area to help the medication absorb better and reduce soreness. Apply a warm compress to ease any stiffness or tenderness. You can add the warm compress before you start feeling sore, right after your injection. It will help the medication absorb faster and reduce hard lumps.

Pro Tip: Switch up your injection sites regularly to avoid irritation or lumps. You can discuss different injection sites with your doctor. Also test the different sites and find places where you experience the least discomfort.

8. Fatigue (Progesterone, Steroids)

Fatigue is common due to the hormonal changes induced by progesterone and steroids.

Tip: Power Snack

"When you need a pick-me-up, go for a snack that packs a punch!" Keep energy-boosting snacks like Nut Butter & Banana Bites, or a trail mix of mixed nuts and dried fruit, on hand to keep your energy levels stable throughout the day.

Pro Tip: Incorporate mini-breaks throughout your day to rest. A quick 5-10 minute break can make a huge difference in recharging your batteries. Don't overdo it during this time. Be selfish with your time. For a couple of weeks try focusing on yourself, your mental health and the process.

9. Antibiotic Side Effects (Supporting Medications)

Antibiotics used during IVF can sometimes lead to gastrointestinal issues, yeast infections, or skin rashes.

Tip: Probiotics for Gut Health

"Give your gut some love!" Add probiotics to your diet to balance your digestive system. Snack on yogurt with fresh fruit or consider a probiotic supplement to keep your stomach in check during antibiotic treatment. Don't eat food that you know upsets your stomach and water, water and more water is your best friend during this time.

Pro Tip: Stay hydrated and drink plenty of water to flush out toxins. If you experience signs of infection or discomfort, don't wait—contact your healthcare provider right away.

Guidance on When to Consult a Healthcare Provider

While most side effects of IVF medications are manageable and temporary, some require medical attention. Here's a quick guide on when to contact your healthcare provider:

1. Severe Abdominal Pain or Cramps

If you experience severe abdominal pain, particularly after taking hCG, it could be a sign of ovarian hyperstimulation syndrome (OHSS) or another serious issue. Don't wait to contact your doctor if the pain is intense or accompanied by bloating and nausea, do so immediately. Put yourself first and make sure to stay on top of things.

2. Difficulty Breathing or Chest Pain

If you experience shortness of breath, chest pain, or swelling in your legs, contact your healthcare provider immediately. These could be signs of a blood clot or other serious complications. Monitor your body closely.

3. Unusual Bleeding or Spotting

While mild spotting can occur in IVF, and can be completely normal, heavy bleeding or blood clots should be evaluated by your doctor to rule out any potential problems.

4. Persistent or Severe Side Effects

If side effects such as nausea, headaches, or fatigue do not improve after a few days, or if they become severe and affect your mental health in a serious way, it's essential to consult with your healthcare provider. Your physical and mental health walk hand in hand, if the one stumbles, so does the other.

5. Emotional Well-Being

IVF can take a toll on your emotional health. If you experience depression, anxiety, or overwhelming feelings, seek support from a mental health professional. IVF-related stress and hormonal changes can sometimes contribute to emotional difficulties, and there's no shame in asking for help. Remember that your hormones are a bit over the place, experiencing unusual emotional feelings is normal, but it is very important to stay on top of things, monitor your emotional well-being. Join IVF communities on facebook, share your story, reach out to family or friends and stay connected to those around you.

Common Side Effects Management Table:

Medication	Common Side Effects	Management Tips	When to Consult a Healthcare Provider
Hormonal Medications (FSH, LH, GnRH)	Hot flashes, mood swings, headaches, bloating, weight gain	Stay cool, hydrate, practice mindfulness, exercise	Severe mood swings, excessive bloating, prolonged headaches
hCG (Human Chorionic Gonadotropin)	OHSS, abdominal pain/cramps, nausea	Stay hydrated, monitor symptoms, gentle movement	Severe pain, difficulty breathing, excessive swelling
Progesterone	Injection site reactions, bloating, fatigue	Rotate injection sites, massage the area, stay active	Pain at the injection site not subsiding, severe bloating

| Supporting Medications (Steroids, Antibiotics, Thyroid Medications) | Weight gain, fatigue, gastrointestinal distress, skin reactions | Eat balanced meals, stay active, take medication with food when possible | Prolonged side effects, unusual rashes, or digestive issues |

Frequency of Common Side Effects from IVF Medications

This bar chart illustrates the prevalence of common side effects experienced by individuals undergoing IVF treatment. The chart highlights how frequently certain side effects, such as mood swings, nausea, and bloating, occur, helping you understand what to expect during your IVF journey.

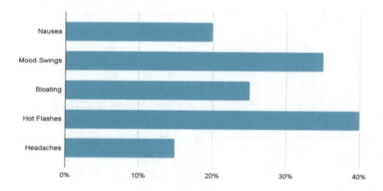

Conclusion

In this chapter we have covered all you need to know about the side effects that accompany IVF. The presence of side effects in IVF medication is common, yet they can be managed efficiently with appropriate approaches. I believe the tips and tricks on managing side effects will help you as much as it did me. Taking a proactive approach to managing side effects during the IVF process, such as staying hydrated, journalling, connecting with support groups, massaging, applying warm compresses and contacting healthcare providers for severe symptoms, can help you feel more in control and alleviate the discomfort. Remember: Take care of your body and it will take care of you.

"The road to conception is one of resilience, where every challenge faced and every dose administered carries you closer to the dream you're nurturing."

Chapter 6: Customizing Your Medication Protocol

Introduction to Personalized IVF Treatment Plans

When it comes to IVF, there's no one-size-fits-all approach. That is what makes this process so amazing. It is specifically designed for you. Just like your fertility journey is unique, so too should your medication protocol be. Personalizing your treatment plan is a crucial step in maximizing your chances of success and ensuring the process works best for your body.

Each woman's response to IVF medications can be different, and your healthcare team will carefully design your medication protocol based on various factors that affect how your body will react to treatment. Since women from all walks of life, all ages and all medical histories try out IVF, the protocols need to be adjusted and tweaked to fit everyones needs perfectly. This chapter explores how IVF medications are tailored to your individual needs, and why understanding the process is vital to get the most out of the process.

Why Personalized Medication Protocols Matter

A customized medication plan helps ensure that each stage of IVF — from stimulating your ovaries to supporting your pregnancy — goes smoothly. Tailored protocols are important because they:

- **Maximize Your Chances:** By adjusting medications to suit your body, doctors can increase the likelihood of a successful IVF cycle.
- **Reduce Risks:** Personalized treatment plans help minimize side effects and complications, such as ovarian hyperstimulation syndrome (OHSS).

- **Address Underlying Issues:** Whether you have conditions like PCOS, endometriosis, or unexplained infertility, your treatment can be adjusted to target your specific needs.

Factors That Influence Your IVF Medication Protocol

Infertility is caused by many different factors and therefore it is important to take into consideration all the possible reasons in combination with your medical history. Your healthcare team will consider several factors when customizing your IVF protocol. These include your age, diagnosis, and your overall health. Here's a look at how these elements come into play:

Age

- Younger women (under 35) often have more eggs available for retrieval, meaning medications that stimulate the ovaries may be used at lower doses.
- Women over 35 may require stronger doses of medication or a different mix of drugs to help stimulate more follicles. As age increases, egg quality can decrease, which might influence the type of medications needed.

Diagnosis

- Polycystic Ovary Syndrome (PCOS): Women with PCOS may be prescribed medications like gonadotropins to stimulate multiple follicles, but doses will be carefully adjusted to avoid OHSS.
- Endometriosis: For those with endometriosis, a combination of GnRH agonists/antagonists may be used to suppress hormone production and prevent ovarian cysts from forming.
- Low Ovarian Reserve: Women with lower egg counts might require medications like hCG or growth hormone to encourage the ovaries to produce more eggs.

Previous IVF History

- If you've undergone IVF before, your healthcare provider will consider how your body responded to previous cycles and adjust medications accordingly.

Tips for Discussing Your IVF Medication Protocol

It's important to feel involved in the decisions about your medication plan. It is your body so you need to feel free to speak up if you don't agree with certain protocols or if you don't respond well to certain medications. Many women feel they need to suffer in order to succeed and that is not the truth. Remember that you need to be healthy in order for the baby to be healthy, you need to be happy in order for the baby to be happy. So if your body is not responding well to medications and it is influencing your mental health in a drastic way you need to make these concerns known. You need to be happy and healthy to give your little one the best chance at success. Here are a few tips to help you have a productive conversation with your healthcare team:

Be Open and Honest About Your Health History

Your doctor needs to know as much as possible about your fertility history, conditions (like PCOS or endometriosis), lifestyle, and previous IVF cycles. This will help them make informed decisions about the best protocol for you. I live by this principle when it comes to appointments: "If you can remember it, mention it." If there is something in your medical history no matter how small that you can remember, mention it. It might give the doctor some insights that you didn't think it would.

Ask Questions

Don't hesitate to ask your doctor why they recommend certain medications or doses. Understanding the rationale behind your protocol will help you feel more in control and the process will make more sense. Some good questions include:
- "What medications will I be taking and why?"
- "What are the potential side effects of each medication?"
- "How will my protocol change if we have to adjust it during the cycle?"
- "What do women complain about when it comes to this medication?"
- "Why do you think this is the best fit for me?"

Discuss Medication Timing

Make sure you understand when and how each medication needs to be taken. Ask for a clear schedule and checklist, and make sure you know how to handle missed doses or changes in your treatment plan. Use the medication tracker in chapter 1 to fill in your schedule immediately.

Inquire About Alternatives

If you're concerned about the medications being prescribed, ask your doctor if there are alternatives or options to manage potential side effects. They may be able to modify your plan or offer options that make you more comfortable. Also remember to always remind doctors of any allergies, no matter how small and insignificant you think it might be.

How Your IVF Medication Protocol is Customized

This table outlines the process of how your healthcare team customizes your IVF medication protocol. Each step is carefully tailored to your unique health needs, diagnosis, and response during the cycle, ensuring a personalized approach to your fertility journey.

Step	Action	Description
Step 1	Assess Your Health History	Review factors like age, diagnosis, lifestyle, and previous IVF cycles.
Step 2	Diagnose & Determine Medication Needs	Based on your health condition (PCOS, endometriosis, etc.), the doctor will determine appropriate medications.
Step 3	Choose Medication Protocol	Select medications like ovarian stimulants (FSH), GnRH agonists, hCG, and progesterone, depending on your needs.
Step 4	Adjust Protocol (if needed)	Modify medication doses or switch medications based on your response during the cycle.
Step 5	Monitor Progress	Regular blood tests and ultrasounds to track the response to medication and adjust doses.

Sample IVF Medication Protocol

Here's an example of how a typical IVF medication protocol might be tailored for different scenarios:

Factor	Personalized Protocol
Age: Under 35	Lower doses of ovarian stimulants (e.g., FSH) to avoid overstimulation.
Age: Over 35	Higher doses of ovarian stimulants, possibly combined with growth hormone.
PCOS Diagnosis	Gonadotropins to stimulate multiple follicles, with careful monitoring to avoid OHSS.
Endometriosis Diagnosis	GnRH agonists to suppress ovarian cysts and enhance egg quality.

Conclusion

One of the amazing aspects of IVF is the ability to customize. Your whole history is taken into consideration when this process is planned and that makes it a true scientific marvel. Personalized IVF treatment plans are key to optimizing your chances of success. By working closely with your healthcare team and understanding the factors that influence your protocol, you can feel confident that your medications are chosen with your specific needs in mind. By asking questions and understanding the process you are able to take your shots with determination and understanding. Take an active role in the conversation, ask questions, and keep track of your treatment progress. Be active, take notes, this is such a special process even though it might feel overwhelming.

"Just as the body needs care to create life, so too does the heart need reassurance. Trust in the process, for every step brings you closer to the possibility of tomorrow."

Chapter 7: Effective Medication Management Strategies

Managing IVF medications can feel overwhelming at times, but with a little organization and the right strategies, you can take control of your medication schedule and reduce the stress that comes with it. We have talked before about your first and second brain. This is a key concept when it comes to IVF. Use your first brain only for the less important things, don't cloud your mind with a million to-do lists and a thousand tasks that need attention. Your mind should be decluttered and you can do this by using apps on your phone or even just your calendar or note app to write down anything that comes up during the day or during your appointments. "I need to inject myself each morning at 8 o'clock, before breakfast." Write it down, set an alarm for each morning at 8 o'clock. You don't need to remember it, your alarm will remind you. Take a few seconds and set the reminder, because you will be set up for the coming weeks and not miss any doses. Your second mind can be cluttered, your phone can do the work. All you have to do is take it easy. IVF requires precise timing and coordination, especially with injectable medications, so having a solid plan in place is key. This chapter will provide practical tips for tracking medications, organizing your administration schedule, and preparing for both injections and oral medications, all while ensuring you maintain peace of mind.

Practical Tips for Tracking Medications and Schedules

Staying on top of your medication schedule is one of the most important parts of IVF. You'll be given a list of medications, each with specific dosages and times for administration. Missing or delaying a dose, especially with medications like hormones or stimulants, can have an impact on your cycle. To make sure you're following the protocol correctly and on time, here are some practical tips:

Create a Medication Calendar

You already have one, you can download the medication Calendar in chapter 1, customize it and make it beautiful if you like, add some color, a picture or two if you want. Make the process beautiful. The first step is to create a visual plan. A medication calendar allows you to see your treatment schedule at a glance. You can use a traditional paper calendar or set up a digital calendar on your phone or computer, where you can input your medication times and doses. I always stick to a digital calendar, because I know the chances of me losing it is far less than a paper alternative.

Tip: Color-code the calendar to differentiate between oral medications, injectables, and any other forms of treatment (like patches). This visual cue can be incredibly helpful to avoid confusion.

Pro Tip: Many IVF clinics provide patients with a medication calendar upon starting treatment. Be sure to review this calendar with your doctor to ensure it's complete and accurate.

Your phone can be an invaluable tool during this process. Set alarms or reminders for each medication, including the specific time of day and any special instructions (e.g., "Inject in the evening"). Most phones have built-in reminder features,or note apps, and you can find really beautiful apps on the app store as well if you want to level it up a bit. There are also specialized apps designed specifically for medication management. This will ensure you stay on track without worrying about forgetting doses.

Tip: Make your reminders sound distinct from your regular alarms to help trigger the importance of the task.

Tools for Organizing Medication

There are many tools and resources available to help you organize and streamline the process of medication management. Let's look at a few options that can make this process smoother:

Medication Management Apps

Apps designed to help with medication tracking can offer more advanced features than simple reminders. These apps can notify you of missed doses, track multiple medications, and even record side effects. Some apps are also designed to send updates to your healthcare provider about your medication schedule and progress, offering an extra layer of support and communication.

Some popular apps to consider are:

App Name	Features	Available On	Best For
Medisafe	Medication reminders, dose tracking	iOS, Android	General medication management
MyTherapy	Medication tracking, symptom journal	iOS, Android	Tracking multiple health factors
Pillboxie	Visual pill organizer, reminders	iOS	Simple medication reminders

These apps help ensure you're following your protocol correctly and provide an easy way to share information with your healthcare team if needed.

Pill Organizers

For oral medications, pill organizers with compartments for each day or dose can help you stay organized. You can find pill organizers with morning, afternoon, and evening compartments, and some even have separate slots for each day of the week.

For injectables, while a pill organizer may not be practical, a specialized storage box with compartments for each vial or medication kit can help. Keep your injectable medications in a cool, dry place and store them according to the instructions (e.g., in the fridge if necessary).

Preparing for Injections and Oral Medications

One of the most stressful aspects of IVF medications for many women is the injections. But with some preparation and practice, they become much easier to handle. Whether you're taking injections or oral medications, it's essential to be as prepared as possible to avoid unnecessary stress and ensure that you're administering your medication correctly.

Injection Preparation Guide

"I'll admit it—I hate needles. And I'm pretty sure you do too! Whenever I take my son for a shot or a blood test, I tell him not to be scared and put on my brave face. But inside, I'm thinking, *Yikes, that's a big needle!* It's okay to feel a little squeamish—it just means we're human!" This step-by-step guide will help you feel more confident and prepared when administering your IVF injection. Whether you're new to injections or just need a quick refresher, following these steps will make the process easier and safer.

Step	Action	Description
1. Gather Supplies	Syringe, Needle, Medication	Collect everything you'll need: syringe, needle, and prescribed medication.
2. Clean Injection Site	Alcohol Swab	Use an alcohol swab to clean the skin where you'll administer the injection. Let it dry.
3. Fill Syringe	Syringe and Medication	Draw the prescribed medication into the syringe, ensuring there are no air bubbles.
4. Administer Injection	Injection Site	Hold the syringe at a 90° angle, insert the needle, and slowly administer the medication.

| 5. Dispose of Sharps Safely | Sharps Container | Safely dispose of the used syringe and needle in a sharps container. |

Oral Medications: Tips and Preparation

While injections can feel more intimidating, oral medications are simpler to manage but require careful timing. Here are a few tips:

1. Follow Instructions on Timing: For medications taken by mouth, some need to be taken with food, and others on an empty stomach. Be sure to follow the instructions given by your doctor or pharmacist.

2. Use a Pill Organizer: For multiple oral medications, a pill organizer is an excellent way to ensure you don't forget any doses. You can separate your doses by the day, or even by the time of day (morning, noon, evening).

3. Stay Consistent: Take your medications at the same time each day, as consistency helps ensure that the medication works effectively. If you're on a time-sensitive medication (e.g., hCG), try to take it at the same time each day to avoid any variations.

4. Drink Plenty of Water: When taking oral medications, drinking plenty of water is key. Not only does it help with digestion, but it can also help reduce nausea or any discomfort from taking multiple pills.

Conclusion

Effectively managing your IVF medications is vital to your treatment's success, and to your sanity. Staying organized from the get-go makes the biggest difference. By following the tips above like using a medication calendar, setting reminders, and tracking your doses, you'll keep yourself organized and on track. Preparing for injections, using medication management apps or journals, and following a routine for oral medications can help ease the process, ensuring you're ready for each step.

Remember, it's perfectly normal to feel a little anxious or uncertain at times, but the more you familiarize yourself with the process and the tools available to you, the more confident you'll become. Keep open lines of communication with your healthcare team, and don't hesitate to ask questions or seek help when needed.

IVF can be a long and sometimes challenging journey, but with the right strategies in place, to decomplicate and simplify the process you're setting yourself up for success.

"In the quiet moments between injections, remember that you're not just waiting—you're creating, growing, and laying the foundation for something beautiful."

Chapter 8: Additional Resources and Support

The IVF journey is not one you have to navigate alone. I highly recommend that you don't. I know that family and friends can sometimes be our greatest enemies in times of need and you might not feel comfortable talking to them about the process, but remember that there are thousands of women that are going through exactly what you are and most of them would also love a friend. Join support groups, facebook groups or ask your doctor about any groups in the area. Finding the right information and emotional support is just as important as understanding the medications and treatment options involved. Whether you're just beginning your IVF path or are in the thick of it, there are countless resources available to help you feel more informed, supported, and understood.

In this chapter, we'll highlight some of the most reliable resources, including websites, books, support groups, and ways to find credible information about IVF medications. We'll also touch on the importance of maintaining your emotional health throughout this journey, because caring for your mind is just as vital as caring for your body.

1. Resources for IVF Patients: Websites, Books, and Support Groups

Websites

The internet can be a wealth of knowledge, but it's important to find trustworthy sources of information. Here are a few recommended websites for IVF patients that can offer a mix of medical insights, emotional support, and practical advice:

- American Pregnancy Association Website

Offers reliable, science-backed information on IVF and other fertility treatments.
- Resolve: The National Infertility Association Website
A comprehensive support network for people going through infertility, with helpful resources, webinars, and local group connections.
- FertilityFriend Website
A popular site for tracking fertility cycles and learning about IVF treatments, often with interactive tools and resources.

Books
While there are countless books on IVF, we recommend looking for those that offer clear, practical advice with empathy. Here are a few titles that have helped many women on their fertility journeys:

- *The IVF Journey* by Dr. Sally M. Dugan

A compassionate guide that outlines each stage of IVF, from initial consultations to managing medications and monitoring progress.

- The No-BS guide to IVF Egg and Embryo Freezing by Jane Claire Aldridge

A deep dive into embryo freezing and egg preservation. Success rates and processes involved.

- *It Starts with the Egg* by Rebecca Fett

A deep dive into the science of fertility, this book gives actionable advice for improving your egg quality before starting IVF.

- *Infertility Survival Handbook* by Elizabeth Swire Falker

A guide to help couples face the emotional challenges of infertility, with tips for managing stress and communication.

Support Groups Support groups are an essential part of many IVF journeys. Not only do they provide emotional comfort, but they also offer a space for sharing experiences, advice, and coping strategies.

- Resolve Support Groups
  Resolve's support groups are designed to connect you with others facing similar challenges in your area. They provide a great outlet for sharing experiences and emotions.
- Fertility Network UK Website
  Offers online and in-person support groups for women undergoing IVF, as well as access to a team of counselors and coaches.
- Facebook Groups and Forums
  Platforms like Facebook host a variety of private groups dedicated to IVF journeys, including groups for specific treatments, age ranges, and countries. These can be excellent spaces to connect with others, ask questions, and gain perspective on different IVF experiences.

2. Seeking Emotional and Informational Support

The IVF journey can feel overwhelming at times. It's easy to become consumed by medications, appointments, and schedules, but it's essential to nurture your emotional health throughout the process.

Emotional Support

Starting IVF can be an emotional rollercoaster. The highs of hope and anticipation, followed by the lows of disappointment and uncertainty, can feel exhausting. Connecting with others who are going through the same experience, or seeking counseling when needed, can make a world of difference.

Therapists Specializing in Fertility

Talking to a therapist who specializes in fertility can help you work through the emotional aspects of IVF. They can guide you through difficult feelings and help you find ways to cope with the challenges. Websites like [Psychology Today](#) offer directories for finding therapists with specific experience in fertility.

Partner Support

Don't forget to lean on your partner or spouse during this journey. IVF affects both of you, and staying emotionally connected can help strengthen your relationship during challenging times. Communication is key to ensuring you're both on the same page, emotionally and mentally.

Self-Care Tips

Practicing self-care is vital. Meditation, yoga, journaling, and deep breathing exercises can reduce stress and help clear your mind. Keeping a journal to track your thoughts and feelings can help you process emotions as they arise, offering a helpful release for any anxiety or frustration. Drink some expensive tea, go for a walk, paint or cook. Do what makes your heart smile.

Finding Reliable Information on IVF Medications

It's easy to get overwhelmed with the amount of information available about IVF, especially when it comes to the different medications involved. Having reliable sources to turn to will ensure you make the best choices for your health and fertility.

What to Look for in a Reliable Source

When seeking information on IVF medications, make sure the source is credible. Look for content that is written by fertility specialists, IVF clinics, or trusted medical associations. Websites like the American Society for Reproductive Medicine (ASRM) and other peer-reviewed medical journals are excellent starting points.

Here's a quick checklist to evaluate sources:

- Author Credentials: Are the articles written by fertility experts or medical professionals?
- Evidence-Based: Does the information reference scientific studies or guidelines from reputable organizations like the ASRM?
- Clear and Understandable: Is the information easy to follow without unnecessary jargon? Does it offer practical advice, not just technical details?
- Up-to-Date: Check that the information is current. IVF treatment and medications are constantly evolving, so the source should reflect the most recent guidelines.

Visual Resources:

Reliable IVF Information Sources

Resource	Type	Details
American Society for Reproductive Medicine	Website	Offers evidence-based guidelines on IVF medications and procedures.
Resolve: The National Infertility Association	Support Group/Website	Provides emotional support, resources, and education for IVF patients.
Fertility Friend	Website/Tracking Tool	Tracks fertility cycles and IVF treatments, with a wealth of educational

		articles.
The IVF Journey	Book	A practical guide for IVF patients. Includes insights into managing medications.

Conclusion

Embarking on the IVF journey can be a transformative and emotional experience. You are going to cry, laugh, scream, dance, jump and swear. And that is the beauty of life and creating it. The raw real emotions that only humans can feel and understand. While you might feel overwhelmed and crazy at times, remember how incredible what you are doing truly is. Give yourself credit, realise your courage and then live and swim through the emotions. My father told me many times while growing up: "Sometimes pain just has to be pain and sometimes joy just has to be joy." Embrace it and work through it, embrace it and enjoy it. For you my friend is creating life, life that will also experience the raw emotions of being human. The support you seek, both informational and emotional, is crucial to navigating this challenging path. Whether you're accessing credible information, joining support groups, or taking care of your emotional health, every step you take towards building your support system is a step towards success.

"Patience is not passive; it's the courage to keep moving forward, even when the path ahead is unclear."

Conclusion

As we reach the end of this journey, I believe it's very important to reflect on all that we have learned together. You've embarked upon a journey which seemed to be scary, overwhelming and confusing, but I believe that you have learned a lot and that all the medical confusion seems like grade 1 math now. IVF is a complex and emotional process, but with the right understanding, planning, and support, you are better equipped to face the challenges and triumphs ahead. My thoughts are with you during this journey. May you find all the peace that you yearn for, may all your dreams come true and may your family grow and thrive.

Throughout this book, we've discussed the many facets of IVF— from understanding the medications, to creating personalized treatment protocols and managing your IVF medications with confidence. You now have a clearer picture of how IVF medications work, how to track and manage them, and how to find the support you need for both your physical and emotional health. Let's have a look at all you have learned.

Key Takeaways:

1. Understanding Medications: You've learned about the different categories of IVF medications— from hormonal medications like GnRH Agonists to ovarian stimulants like FSH, and supporting medications like antibiotics and steroids. Knowing what each medication does and how to manage them is crucial for your success.
2. Personalized Protocols: Every IVF journey is unique. Your treatment plan should be customized based on your age, diagnosis, and response to previous treatments. The flexibility in IVF medication protocols ensures that your healthcare team can adjust your treatment for the best possible outcome.
3. Tracking and Managing Your Medications: Keeping track of your medication schedule can be daunting, but it's essential. Tools like apps, medication journals, and simple schedules can help ensure you stay on track and reduce stress.

4. Emotional and Informational Support: IVF is not just a physical process— it's emotional too. Finding the right support system, whether through support groups, therapy, or simply leaning on a trusted friend, is just as important as understanding your treatment.
5. Proactive Self-Care: Don't forget about your mental health. Practicing self-care and seeking emotional support will help you stay resilient through the ups and downs of IVF.

Encouragement for the IVF Journey:

No matter where you are in your IVF journey, please remember—you are not alone. I realise now that I am not alone either. I have you, reading this book. Someone I can share my process with, someone that can hear my story too. So thank you, thank you for giving me the opportunity to share my story, my tears and my triumphs and don't be afraid to share yours too. You might just be the bit of encouragement or the friend that another woman needs desperately right now. Every step you take, from your first consultation to the final outcome, is a part of your very own special story. The story might seem full of uncertainty, but it's also full of possibility. By taking this step, you've already shown incredible strength, and that courage is the exact characteristic that makes GREAT MOTHERS.

Yes, there will be challenges, but there will also be moments of triumph. Every visit to the clinic, every dose of medication, every emotional hurdle you overcome—these are all small victories that bring you closer to your dream of expanding your family. Celebrate those victories, no matter how small they may seem, and remember to take care of yourself—physically, mentally, and emotionally—through it all. You're doing something truly amazing.

Final Thoughts on the Importance of Knowledge and Support:

IVF can sometimes feel like a daunting, complicated journey, but knowledge and support make all the difference. This book has aimed to provide you with clear, factual information, helpful tools, and emotional encouragement, but the most important thing is to never stop asking questions and seeking out the help you need.

Be proactive about your health, engage with your healthcare team, and find the resources that resonate with you. Don't hesitate to reach out for help—whether it's a support group, a trusted friend, or a mental health professional. You deserve the support that will help you feel empowered every step of the way.

As you move forward, remember that this is your journey, and you are in control. Trust in your strength, lean on your support network, and know that there is a path forward, whatever that path may look like.

Stay resilient, stay hopeful, and above all—stay compassionate with yourself. The IVF journey is not just about reaching an end goal; it's about growing through each step and finding strength in every challenge you overcome.

Good luck on your journey—may it be filled with success, hope, and the support you need.

Go kick some ass mama!

"The road to healing is often winding, but every turn brings you closer to the life you're working so hard to create."

Appendix

As you navigate your IVF journey, having a clear understanding of the terms, schedules, and resources related to IVF medications can make the process more manageable. This appendix serves as a helpful reference to support you in your journey, providing essential term definitions and additional resources for further reading.

Glossary of Common IVF Medication Terms

Understanding the terminology used in IVF can help you feel more confident and informed when discussing your treatment with your healthcare team. Below are some common terms you may encounter:

- GnRH Agonists (Gonadotropin-Releasing Hormone Agonists): Medications used to control the release of hormones from the pituitary gland, typically used to suppress ovulation or manage ovarian stimulation.
- GnRH Antagonists: Medications that prevent the premature release of eggs during IVF, typically used alongside ovarian stimulation.
- FSH (Follicle-Stimulating Hormone): A hormone that stimulates the ovaries to produce follicles, which contain eggs. It is often used in IVF to promote the development of multiple eggs.
- hCG (Human Chorionic Gonadotropin): A hormone used to trigger ovulation when eggs are ready for retrieval. hCG also helps support early pregnancy.
- Progesterone: A hormone that helps prepare the uterine lining for implantation and supports early pregnancy following embryo transfer.
- Ovarian Stimulation: The process of using hormones to stimulate the ovaries to produce multiple eggs for IVF, often using medications like FSH and LH.
- Trigger Shot: The final injection (often hCG) given to induce ovulation, signaling that the eggs are ready for retrieval.
- Embryo Transfer: The procedure in which embryos are placed into the uterus following fertilization, aiming for pregnancy.

- Embryo Freezing: The process of preserving embryos for future use, often after an IVF cycle.

References for Further Reading

As you continue your IVF journey, it's important to stay informed about the latest research, developments, and support options. Here are some trusted resources for further reading:

- **Books:**
    - "The No-BS guide to IVF Success rates" Jane Claire Aldridge
    - "Taking Charge of Your Fertility" by Toni Weschler
    - "The Infertility Cure: The Ancient Chinese Medicine Way to Enhance Fertility and Improve Your Odds of Getting Pregnant" by Randine Lewis
    - "The IVF Gift" by Jane Kelwin (A heartfelt journal and guide with digital playlists)
- **Websites:**
    - [American Society for Reproductive Medicine (ASRM)](#) – Offers comprehensive resources on IVF, fertility treatments, and patient support.
    - [The IVF Journey](#) – A supportive community for IVF patients, with forums, articles, and personal stories.
    - [Resolve: The National Infertility Association](#) – A nonprofit organization providing resources for individuals and couples struggling with infertility.
- **Support Groups:**
    - Local and online IVF support groups can provide emotional and practical support. Websites like Facebook, Reddit, and Fertility Network UK host active communities of IVF patients who share experiences and advice.
- **Articles and Journals:**
    - "Recent Advances in IVF Technology" in *Human Reproduction Update*
    - "Psychological Support for IVF Patients: A Literature Review" in *Fertility and Sterility*

Remember, the more informed you are, the better equipped you'll be to navigate the IVF journey and make decisions that are best for you.

This appendix provides the essential tools and resources you need to move forward with confidence. Whether it's keeping track of your medication schedule, learning more about IVF terminology, or seeking out further reading, you're now armed with the knowledge to make empowered choices on your IVF journey.

Disclaimer

This book provides general information about IVF medications based on research and personal insights. It is not intended to replace professional medical advice, diagnosis, or treatment. Always consult with a qualified healthcare provider regarding any questions or concerns about your specific health needs, medications, or fertility treatment options. The author and publisher disclaim any liability for outcomes, reactions, or consequences arising from the use of information in this book. Readers are strongly encouraged to make healthcare decisions in consultation with their medical team.

About the Author

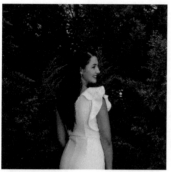

Jane Claire Aldridge is a dedicated author and fertility advocate, combining her chemistry background with a compassionate, approachable writing style to simplify the complexities of IVF for women. Having personally navigated the emotional and scientific challenges of infertility, Jane understands the need for accessible, clear, and empowering information.

With a focus on demystifying IVF, Jane's books present scientific concepts in an easy-to-understand way, without overwhelming readers with technical jargon. Her works, including *The No-BS Guide to IVF Alternatives*, *The No-BS Guide to Egg and Embryo Freezing*, and *The No-BS Guide to IVF Success Rates*, aim to provide women with not only the facts they need but also the emotional support they deserve throughout their fertility journeys.

Each of Jane's books cuts through the noise of confusing medical information, offering clear, actionable insights and advice. Her writing reflects her deep understanding of both the physical and emotional aspects of fertility treatments, ensuring that every woman feels confident, informed, and supported in making the best decisions for herself.

Jane's approach combines scientific clarity with emotional resilience, helping women feel empowered to navigate their fertility choices, whether that's IVF, egg freezing, or exploring alternative treatments. With Jane's guidance, readers can take control of their journey, armed with knowledge and hope for a successful path forward.

Made in the USA
Columbia, SC
24 November 2024